# Total Hip REPLACEMENT

## It's a Joint Effort

## Contents

This book is only to help you learn and should not be used to replace any of your doctor's advice or treatment.

# Introduction

You and your doctor have decided that you will have hip replacement surgery. Total hip replacement will allow you to move more freely and with more comfort than you do now. Billy Joel and Jane Fonda have both had this surgery and now lead active, normal lives.

This booklet will help you know how your hip joint works and will teach you about the surgery to replace it. You will also learn what to do before and after surgery to make sure you get the greatest benefit from your new hip.

On the inside back cover, there is a list of questions you may wish to ask your doctor.

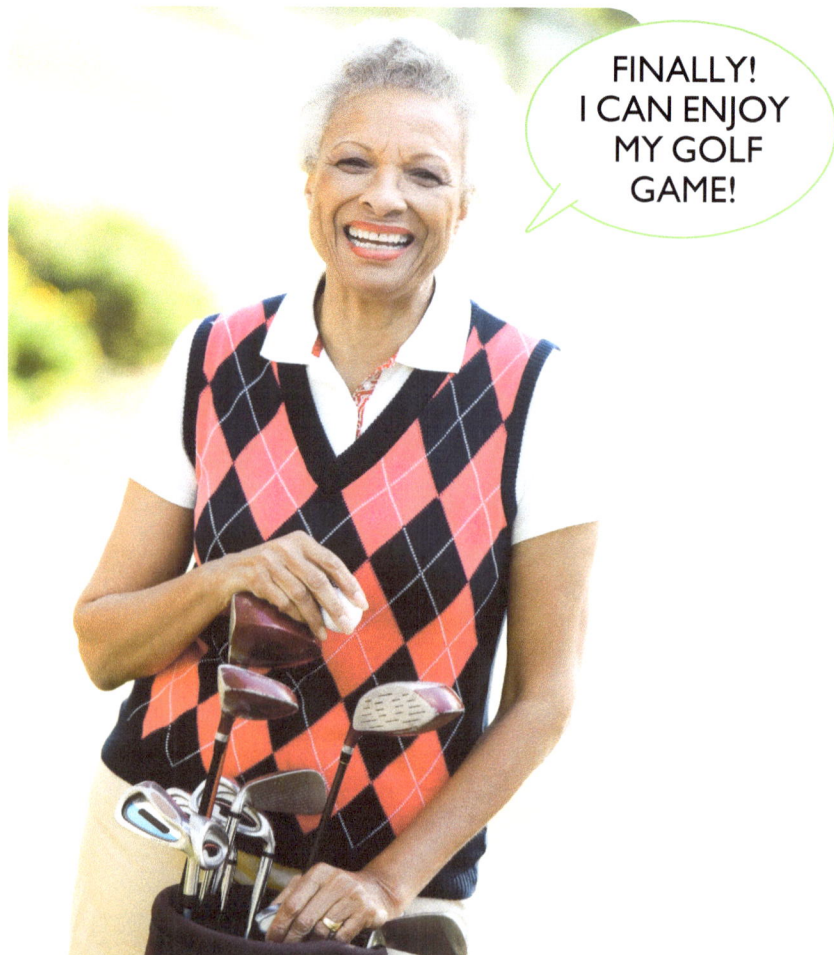

FINALLY! I CAN ENJOY MY GOLF GAME!

# The hipbone's connected to the thighbone

Your hip joint, formed by your thighbone and hipbone, is a ball-and-socket joint. This kind of joint allows the hip to move freely in all directions. Hip joints let you bend over, squat down and pedal a bike. Just think of all the hip movements a gymnast uses in doing a back flip.

The thighbone (femur) is the largest bone in the body. It narrows to a "neck" that points toward the hipbone (pelvis) and ends in a ball-shaped knob (femoral head). This ball is about the size of a golfball and fits into a curved socket (acetabulum) in the pelvis.

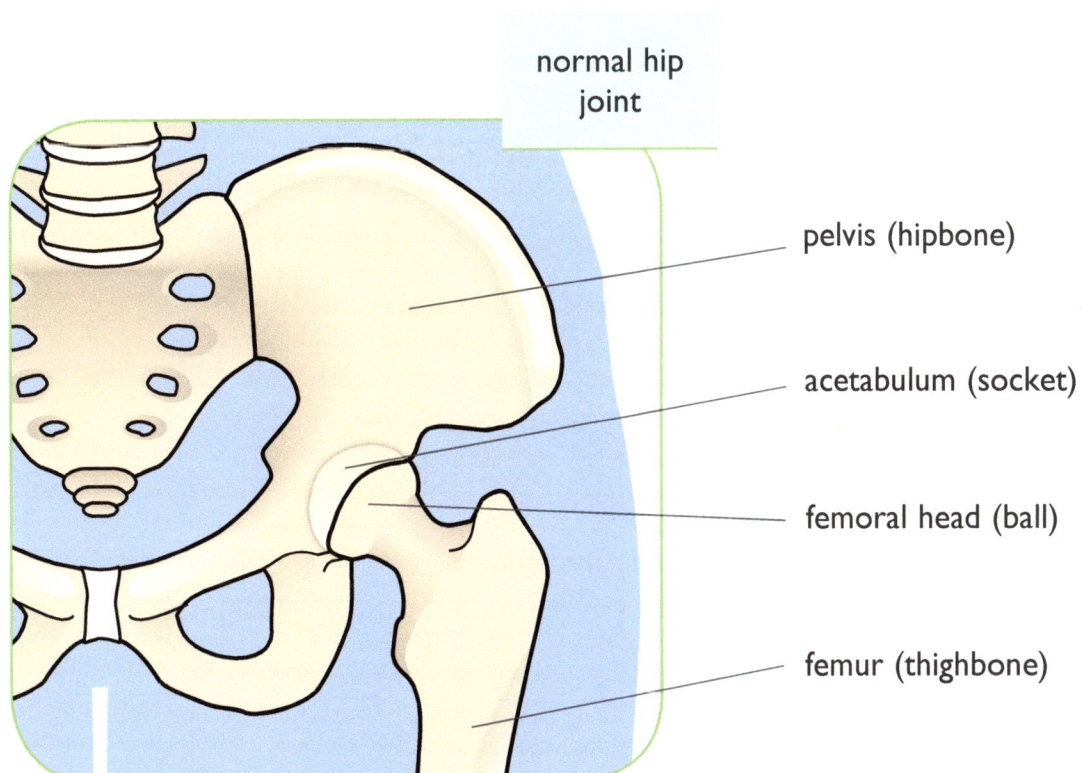

normal hip joint

pelvis (hipbone)

acetabulum (socket)

femoral head (ball)

femur (thighbone)

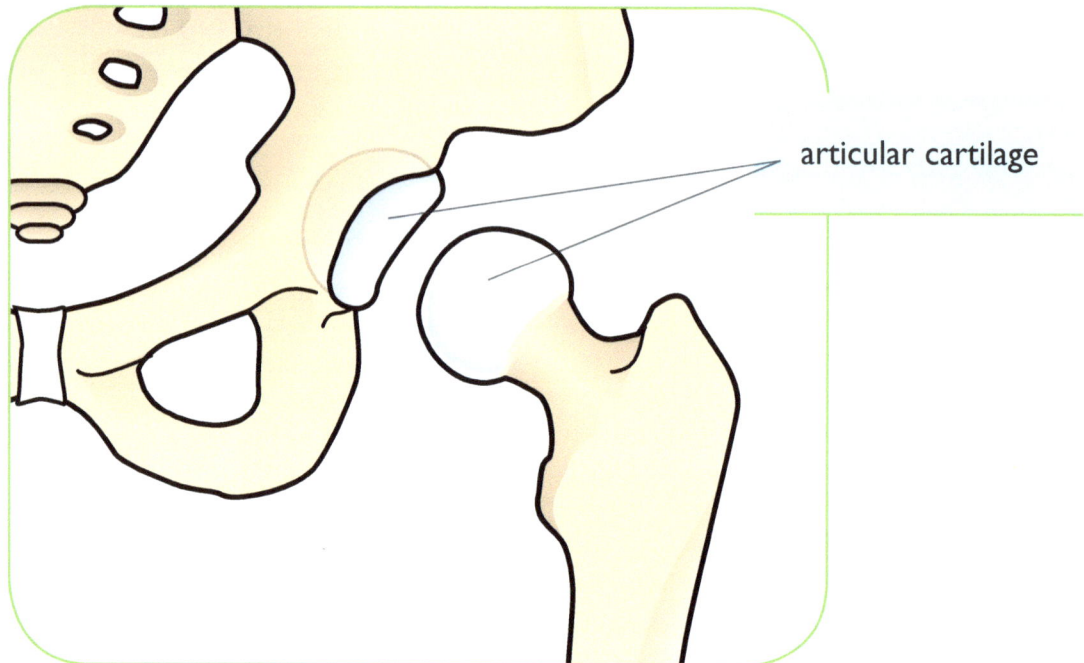

articular cartilage

Without ball-and-socket joints your movements would be stiff, much like a mummy or a robot. (You may have noticed limited motion or stiffness in your hip.)

The large muscles, tendons and ligaments of the thigh and pelvis surround the hip joint. The ligaments and tendons hold the ball and socket in the right position.

A thin membrane (synovial membrane) surrounds the joint. It produces tiny amounts of fluid which lubricate ("oil") the joint. A shiny, smooth substance called articular cartilage covers the ends of the bones. The cartilage provides a smooth surface on your bones that makes movements easy and painless.

# ARTHRITIS

Arthritis is a disease which affects over 43 million people. Arthritis is a "wearing away" of the articular cartilage or joint surface. An injury, disease or normal aging can cause articular cartilage to become thin or worn. When it does, the two bones begin to rub together. This results in painful movements and a slow wearing away of the bone surface.

# ASEPTIC NECROSIS

The ball part of the thighbone gets its blood supply through a small artery. If this artery becomes clogged or injured, the bone will die. This is called avascular or aseptic necrosis (AVN).

# FRACTURE

A broken hip (fracture) is a common injury in people who have osteoporosis. Sometimes the best treatment for the fracture is hip replacement. Other times, the best treatment is fixing the fracture. Osteoporosis, or "soft bone", is common in women after menopause or in men over age 70. The hip most often breaks at the narrow neck of the thighbone.

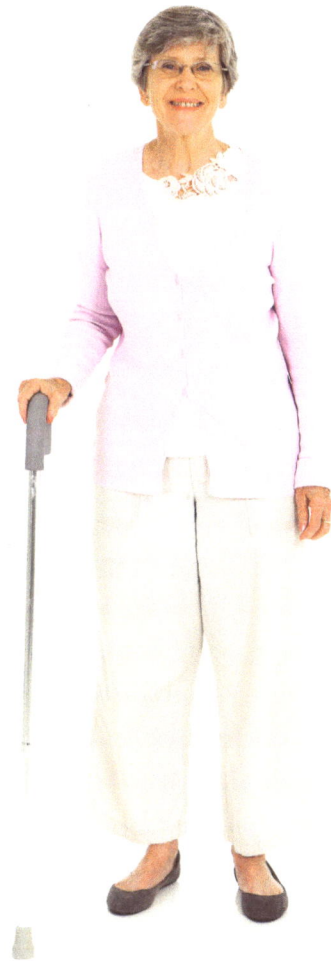

# GETTING YOURSELF READY

Ask your doctor if the hospital offers pre-op classes. A class before surgery can do a lot to help you and your family get ready. Knowing what to expect can help ease your fears, as well.

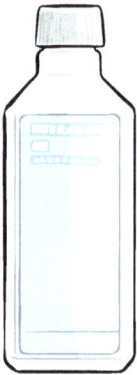

Arrange to have someone stay with you once you are discharged from the hospital.

You will most likely be asked to wash your entire body with a special soap for a number of days before your surgery. The soap is available over-the-counter in many brand names. This will help to prevent infection during your hospital stay.

If you smoke, now is the time to quit! Studies have shown that bones heal much faster in non-smokers.

Talk with your family doctor about your blood levels. You want to have a hgb (hemoglobin) level of over 12 gm/dL. If your level is too low, talk to your doctor about increasing your level by changing your diet.

Here are some other tips to get yourself ready:

- Prepare and freeze meals ahead of time so that you won't have to worry about cooking.

- Think about the room you are going to sleep in. Is it on the same floor as the bathroom and kitchen? If not, is the person caring for you able to carry meals up stairs?

- Put everything you might need on a bedside table so that it will be within easy reach. Make sure to include a phone and a lamp.

- Make sure you are eating a healthy diet and taking any supplements your doctor ordered.

# GETTING YOUR HOUSE READY

Once you have a new hip, you may need to follow some safety rules. This will help you heal faster. Your surgeon will let you know if you have to take special care with your new hip. If you do, one rule is to always sit with your knees lower than your hips. To check around your house, sit:

- on the side of your bed

- in your favorite chair

- on the sofa

- on the toilet

- in the seat of your car

Are your knees always lower than your hips? If not, you can add pillows to any seat and you can buy a raised toilet seat. For other ideas to correct the problem, ask your physical or occupational therapist. Ask a family member to fix the problems before you come home if you don't have time to do it before surgery.

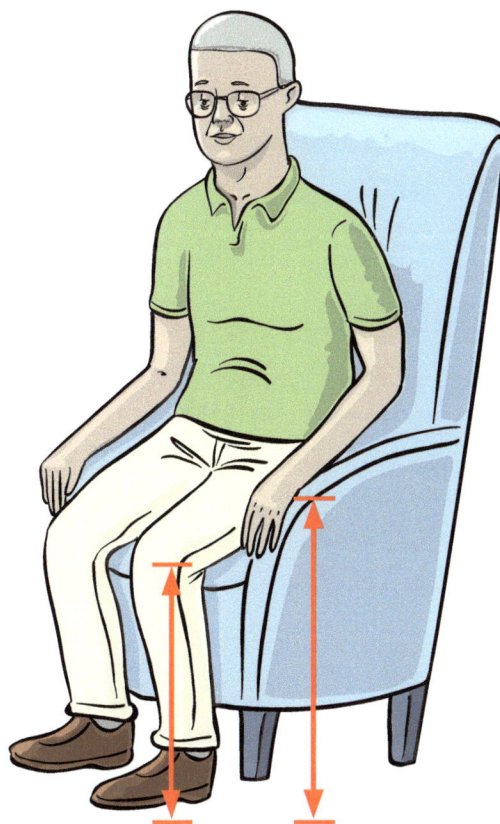

Keep knees lower than hip.

# GETTING READY FOR THE HOSPITAL

When you go to the hospital take these with you:

- [ ] a list of all medicines you take (including over-the-counter)

- [ ] a list of any allergies you have (to food, clothing, medicine, etc.) and how you react to each one

- [ ] glasses, hearing aids and any other items you use each day

- [ ] grooming items such as shampoo, toothpaste, deodorant, etc.

- [ ] loose fitting shoes and shirt to wear for therapy

- [ ] knee length robe or cover-up for walking in the halls

- [ ] shoes with closed in heels and non-slip soles

- [ ] a walker (if you already have one at home)

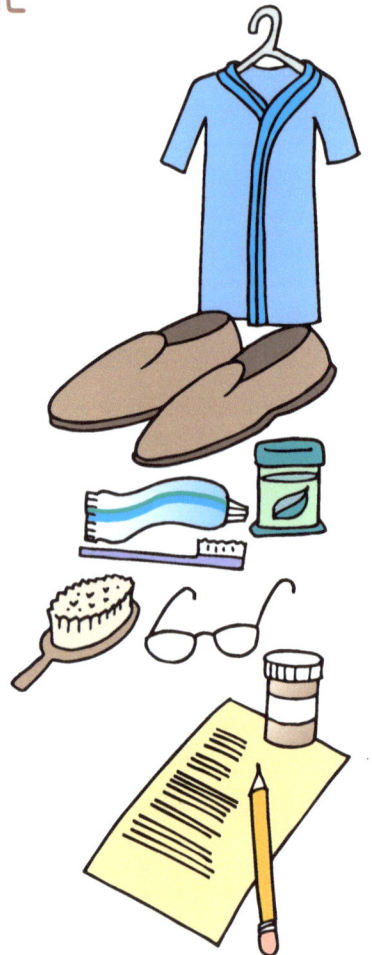

★ Many pain medicines can cause constipation. Prepare now - learn about changes you can make to your diet in case this happens.

★ Put your name on everything you take to the hospital.

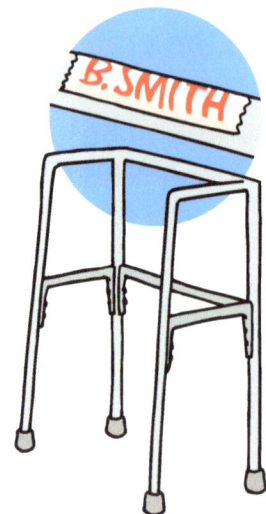

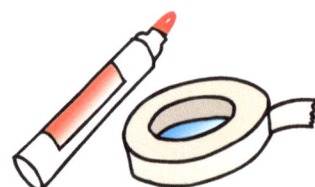

# CONSENT FORM

Before surgery you must sign a consent form. This is a legal paper that says your doctor has told you about your surgery and any risks you are taking. By signing this form, you are saying that you agree to have the operation and know the risks involved. Ask your doctor any questions you may have about the operation and the results before signing this form.

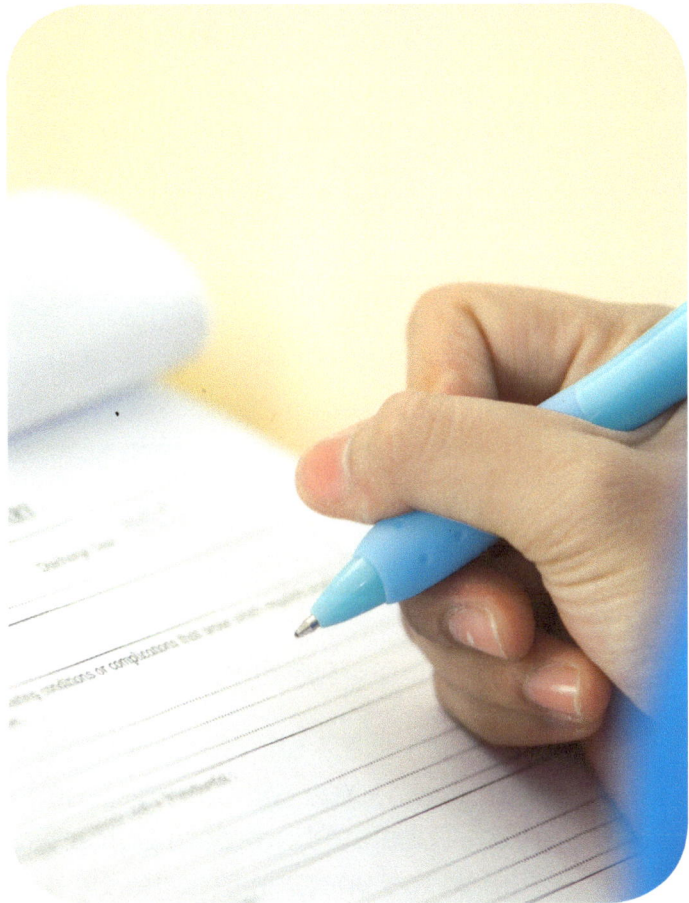

# TESTS BEFORE SURGERY

Most people will have an ECG (heart tracing), a chest X ray and blood tests before surgery. Your orthopaedic surgeon may have you see your family doctor for a checkup. It is important that your blood levels be within a certain range before surgery. Your surgeon will review the results of these tests to make sure you are healthy and ready for surgery.

# THE NIGHT BEFORE SURGERY

Many surgeons prefer that you don't eat or drink after midnight. Check with your doctor or nurse about this. If you take insulin, heart or blood pressure pills on a daily basis, discuss this with your doctor or nurse. They will make sure you do not miss any medicines that you need.

# The morning of surgery

You will be asked to remove:

- dentures, hearing aids

- hairpins, wigs, etc.

- jewelry

- glasses, contact lenses

- nail polish

- all underwear

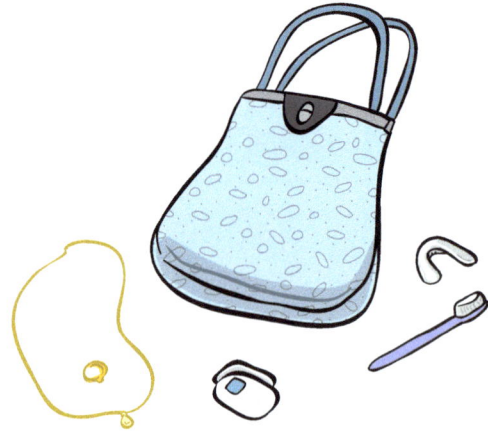

Have your family keep your things for you during surgery.

You will have a short visit with your family before leaving your room.  You will be dressed in a hospital gown (nothing else).  Use the bathroom before you get on the stretcher to ride to the operating room.  Once you are there, your hip will be scrubbed well with a special soap.

After you go to surgery, someone will show your family to the waiting room.  Most of the time, hip surgery lasts from 45 minutes to 2½ hours.  You will also spend some time in the recovery room after surgery, so your time in the surgical area can be as long as 3 to 6 hours.  Your doctor will tell your family about how long you will be away.  From time to time, a member of the surgical team will update your family on your progress.  When the surgery is complete, the doctor will go to the waiting area and give your family a report.

# While you are in surgery

Many people are in the operating room with you. Each hospital has its own routine, but these are some of the people who may be there:

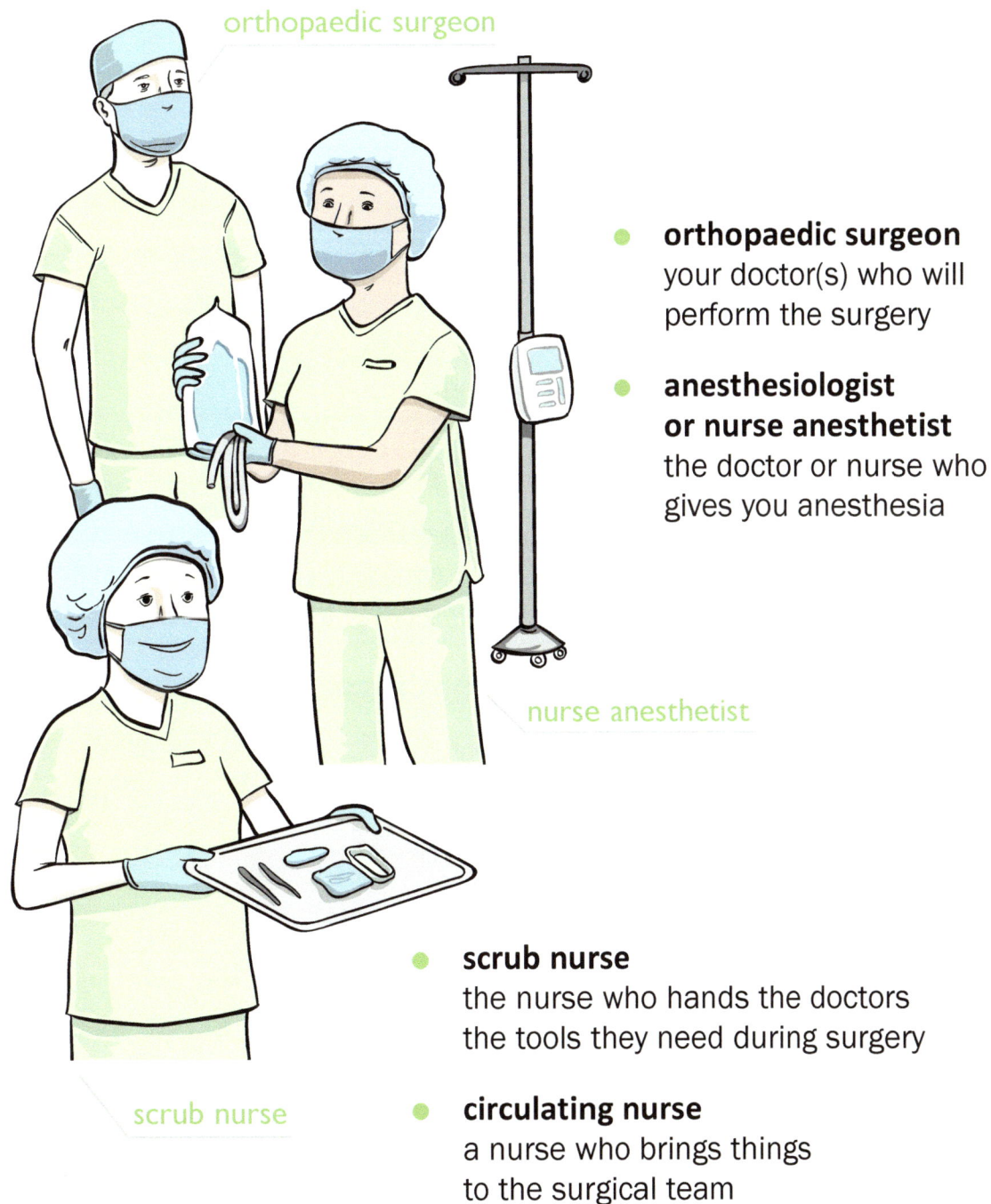

orthopaedic surgeon

nurse anesthetist

scrub nurse

- **orthopaedic surgeon**
  your doctor(s) who will perform the surgery

- **anesthesiologist or nurse anesthetist**
  the doctor or nurse who gives you anesthesia

- **scrub nurse**
  the nurse who hands the doctors the tools they need during surgery

- **circulating nurse**
  a nurse who brings things to the surgical team

Your surgeon and the anesthesiologist or nurse anesthetist will help you choose the best anesthesia to have. No matter what type of anesthesia you have, rest assured that you will not feel pain during the surgery. The types of anesthesia* you may have are:

- **general**
  You are put to sleep.

- **peripheral nerve block**
  Medicine will be injected around the nerves to make part of your body numb. This can be used on surgery for the upper or lower body.

- **epidural**
  You are numbed from the waist down with medicine injected into your back. (This is also used for women giving birth.)

- **spinal**
  Much like epidural, you are numbed from the waist down from medicine injected into your back.

An **intravenous tube (IV)** is placed in your arm. This lets your doctor replace fluids lost during surgery and give you pain medicine, antibiotics and any other medicines you may need.

A **catheter** (tube) may be placed in your **bladder.** This lets your health team keep up with your fluid intake and output. The catheter is most often removed the day after surgery.

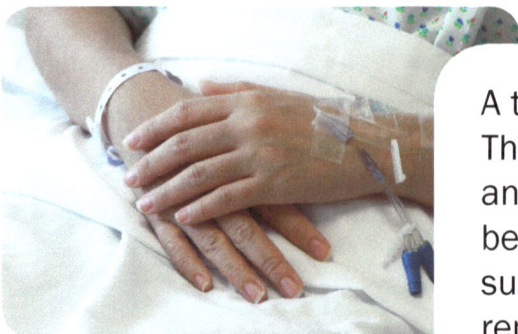

A third tube may come from your bandage site. This is a drain tube that helps reduce blood and fluid buildup at the incision. This tube will be removed as your doctor advises, after your surgery. Most of the time, all tubes will be removed before you leave the hospital.

* Anesthesia may cause nausea. Extreme cases of nausea can be treated with medicine.

# Your new hip

ball
replacement

socket replacement

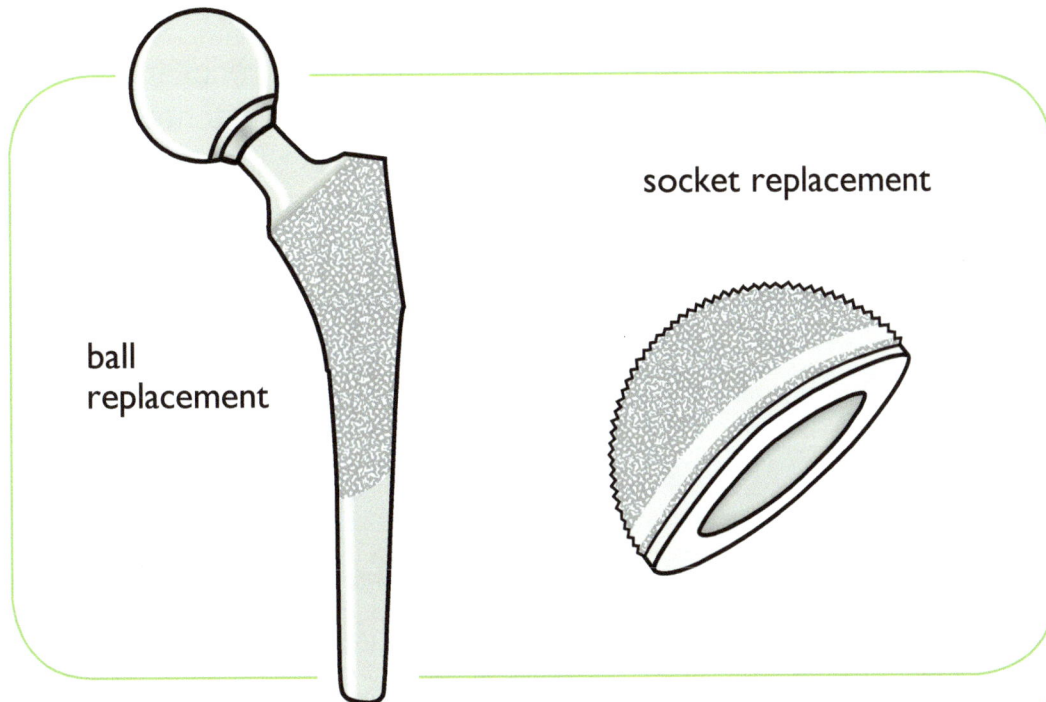

The ball portion of your hip will be removed, and a new metal ball will be put in. The ball part of your new hip has a long stem that allows your doctor to position it firmly into the thighbone.

The socket part of your hip is replaced with a new one that perfectly fits the new ball. The new socket is made of plastic, metal or ceramic. After your surgery is complete, an X ray is made to be sure your hip is in the right position. The incision is closed with stitches or staples, and you are taken to a recovery room.

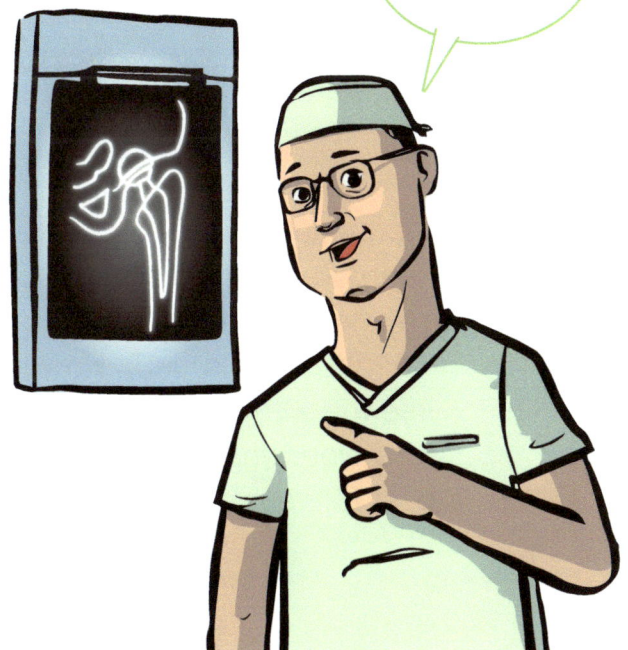

LOOKS GREAT!

# After surgery

## THE RECOVERY ROOM

After surgery,* you will spend a period of time in the recovery room.  Here, your blood pressure and heart rate are watched very closely.  You may have a mask over your face to get oxygen.  Later you will be taken to your hospital room.

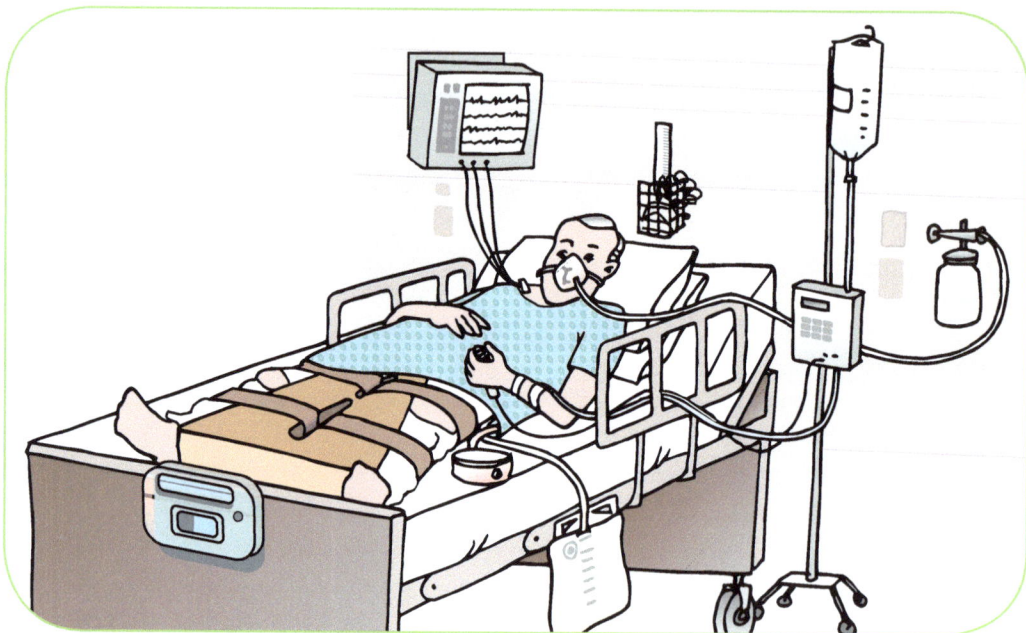

Some doctors will order a V-shaped wedge pillow (abduction pillow) to go between your legs.  This keeps your new hip in the best position. You need to keep this wedge in place when turning in bed.  How long you use the wedge will depend on what your doctor decides is best for you.

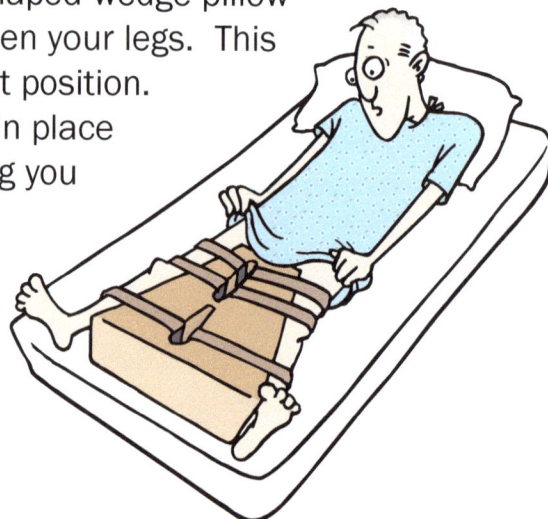

* You may not remember much about the surgery.

# RETURNING TO YOUR HOSPITAL ROOM

## Pain

Talk with your doctor before surgery about your pain medicine options. There are many new medicines and techniques to help you be more comfortable after surgery. You may receive pain medicine through your IV, through the epidural or in shots or pills.

You will most likely experience some pain, but some people have very little. **It is very important that you begin moving around as soon as possible.** To do this you need to manage your pain. Do not wait to tell someone if you are hurting. Waiting may make it harder to relieve the pain. With proper management you can do **exercises and walk.** This is **important to your recovery.**

Your nurse or doctor may use a pain scale to measure the amount of pain you are in. This helps to figure out how well medicines and/or treatments are working. The pain scale may come in the form of a list of numbers, with or without pictures.

Usually, your pain is rated on a scale between 0 and 10, where 0 is no pain and 10 is the strongest pain. Your treatments are adjusted according to the level of pain you are in. So, be honest.

## Pain scale

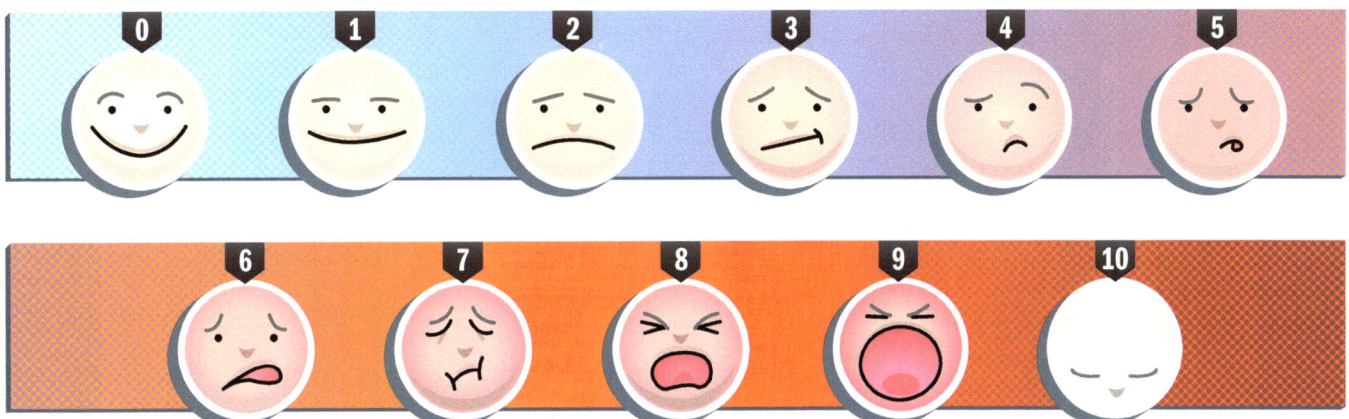

# BREATHING

Right after your surgery, it will seem as if your nurse is always reminding you to take deep breaths and cough. **It is very important that you do this at least every 2 hours.** Deep breathing can help prevent pneumonia or other problems that can slow down your recovery and lengthen your hospital stay.

Your doctor may want you to use a device called an incentive spirometer. This device helps you breathe in and out the right way. Using it regularly and correctly can help keep your lungs clear.

Keep cylinder "floating" as you breathe in

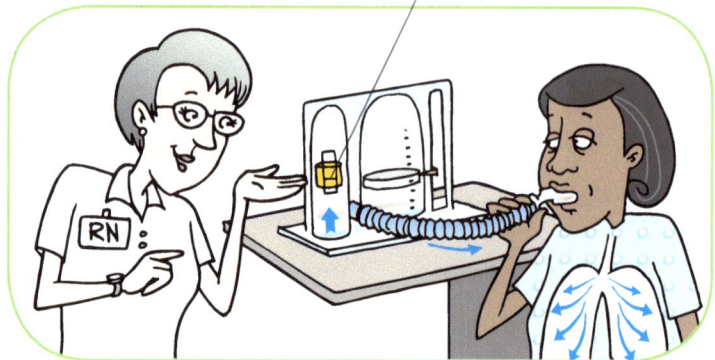

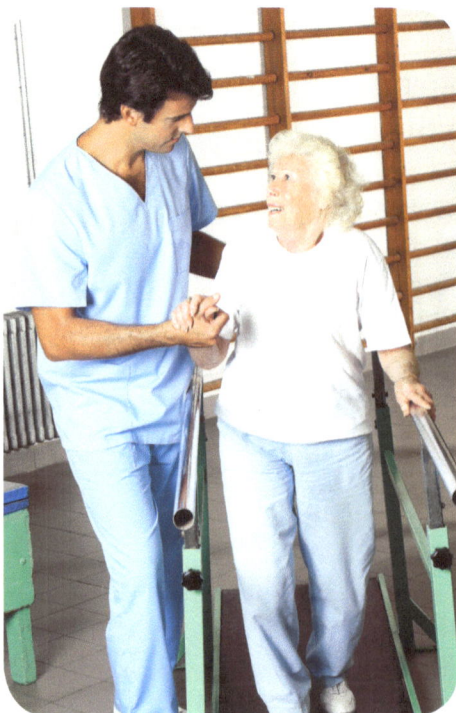

# MOVEMENT

Most people begin exercising their hip the day of, or the day after surgery. A PT will work with you on specific exercises to make your leg and new hip stronger.

# Preventing blood clots

Blood clots are the most common complication after total hip surgery. DVT (deep vein thrombosis) occurs when blood clots form in your abdomen, thigh or calf. If a clot breaks off and goes to your lungs, the blood supply to your lungs is cut off. This is called a pulmonary embolus and can be life-threatening.

The health team will remind you to do foot pumps every hour to push the blood out of your legs. Keep doing these after you go home. You are still at risk for getting blood clots weeks after joint replacement surgery.

**Foot pumps**

Pretend you are pushing down the gas pedal in a car.

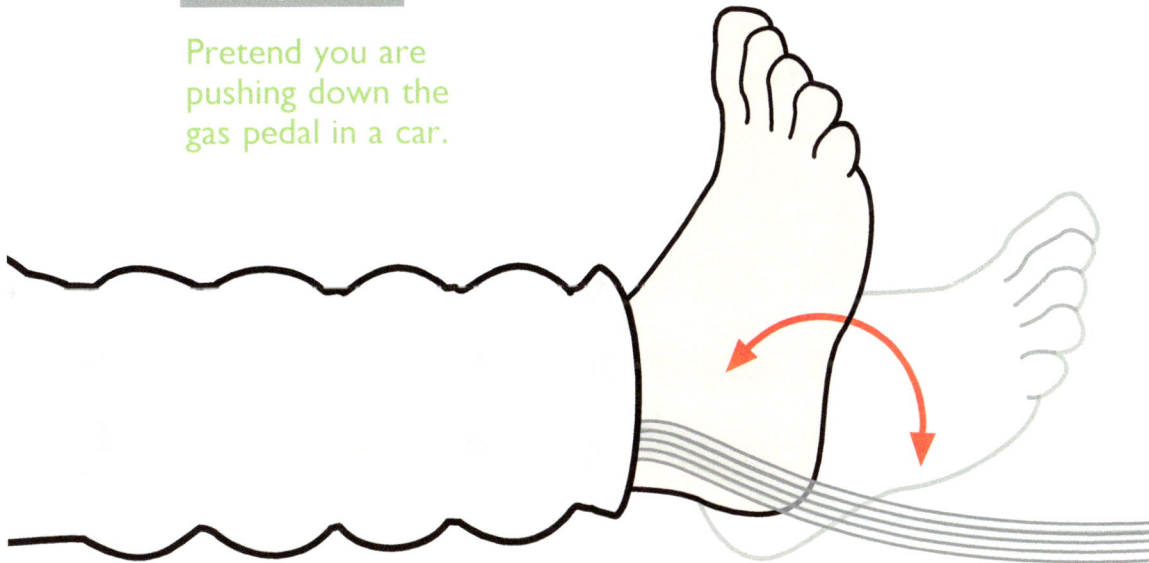

You may have mechanical compression wraps on your legs or feet after surgery. These devices keep the blood from pooling in your legs. Your doctor may also order a blood thinning medicine to reduce the chance of blood clots.

# MOVEMENT (CONTINUED)

Moving around helps prevent DVT after surgery. While you are in the hospital, the health care team will encourage you to get out of bed and walk often. When you go home, it is still very important that you walk often because you are still at risk for DVT for several weeks after surgery.

When sitting, follow any instructions given by your MD or PT. This is to prevent the new ball from popping out of its new socket (dislocation).*

Talk with your nurse or therapist about the right way to get in and out of a car and do tasks such as bathing, dressing and cooking.

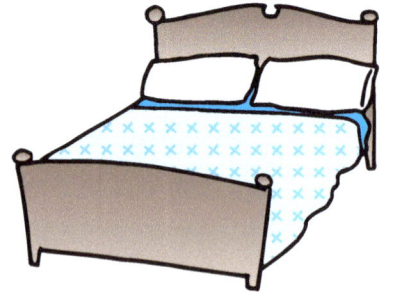

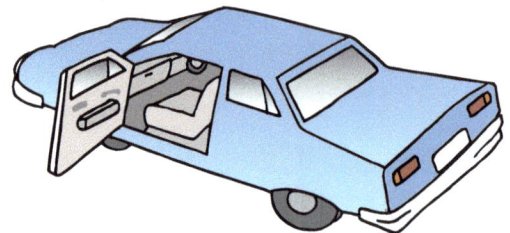

# BEFORE YOU LEAVE THE HOSPITAL

You will learn how to:

- get in and out of bed by yourself

- walk down the hall with your walker or crutches

- get in and out of the shower by yourself

- manage steps at home

- get in and out of your car

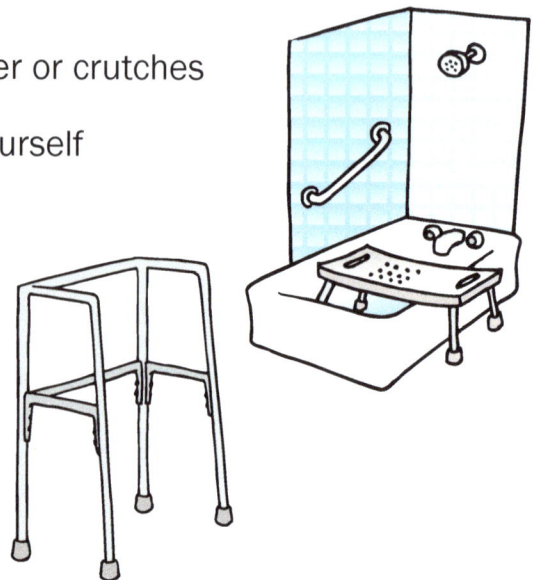

* See the next page for directions on how to prevent hip dislocation.

# Anterior hip precautions
## (if needed)

Depending on your surgery, you may have some safety rules that you need to follow to prevent dislocation of your new hip. Your health team will remind you often of your hip precautions. Ask your doctor how many months you will need to follow these rules after your surgery. **Here are some rules you may be given when your surgery is on the front.**

**DON'T**

. . . stretch your hip back beyond neutral

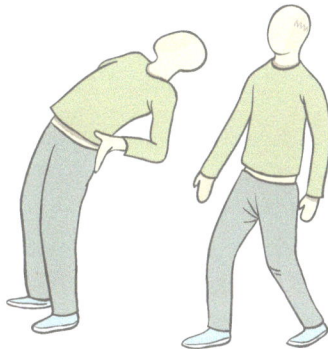

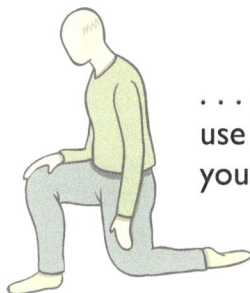

. . . squat down on 1 knee— use both knees to squat or cross your legs

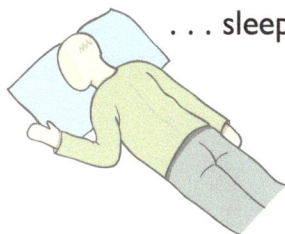

. . . sleep on your stomach

. . . twist upper body away from new hip

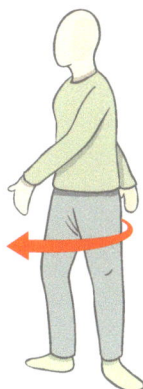

**DO**

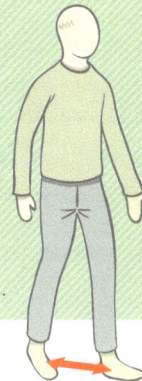

. . . take short steps

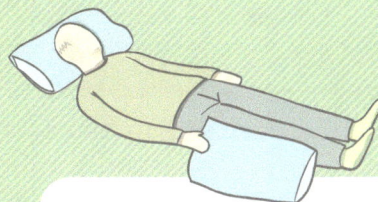

. . . use pillows against your legs and hip at night to keep from rolling on your hip

# Posterior hip precautions
## (if needed)

Depending on your surgery, you may have some safety rules that you need to follow to prevent dislocation of your new hip. Your health team will remind you often of your hip precautions. Ask your doctor how many months you will need to follow these rules after your surgery. **Here are some rules you may be given when your surgery is on the back.**

**DON'T**

bend at your hip past 90°.

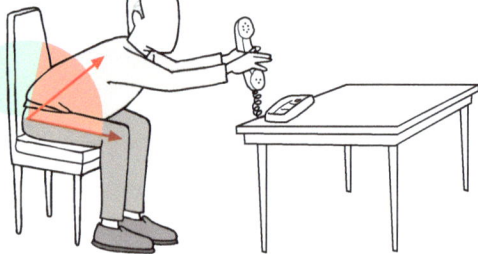

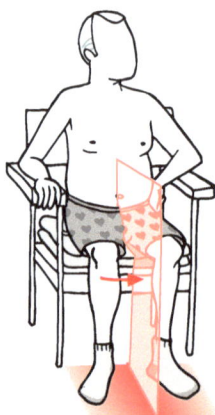

let your knee move inward past your navel.

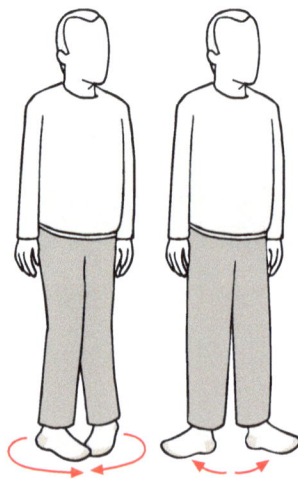

turn your feet in or out.

**DO**

avoid bending more than 90°.

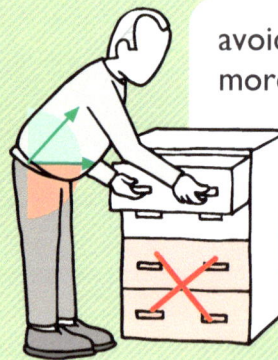

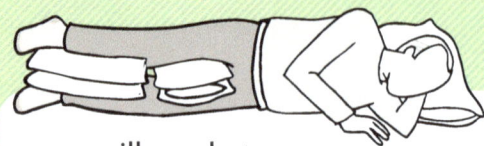

use pillows between your legs at night to keep your hips properly aligned.

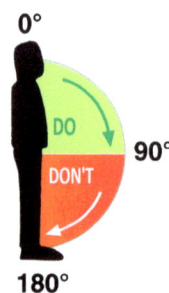

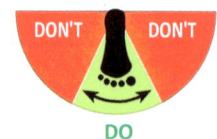

0°

DO

90°

DON'T

180°

DON'T    DON'T

DO

# When you go home

You will be able to leave the hospital in a few days. Your family may need to bring extra pillows for you to sit on in the car. You may find it most comfortable to sit in the front seat of the car. All of the tubes will be out, and a bandage on your hip is all that should remain. If your doctor ordered an abduction wedge, you may still need pillows at night when you are sleeping.

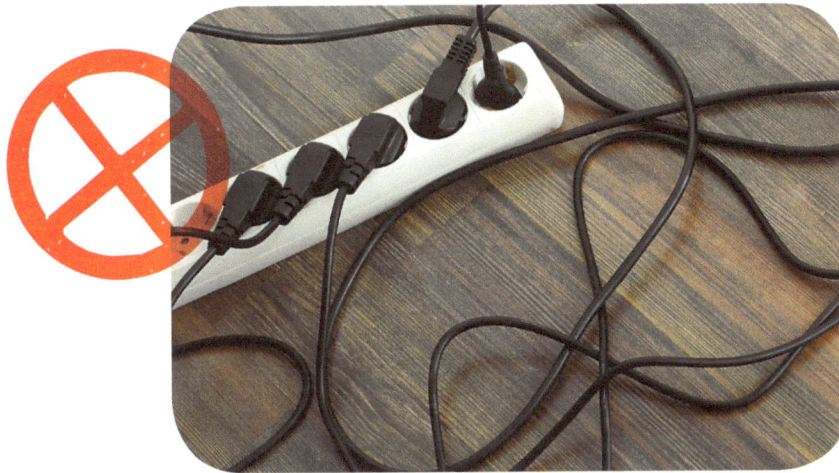

## HOME SAFETY

Special care should be taken when you get home. Some common things in your home may now be a danger to you.

To prevent falls, remove or watch out for:

- long phone or electrical cords that lie across the floor

- loose rugs or carpet

- pets that run in your path

- water spills on bare floors

- wet bathroom tile or slippery floors

- ice or mildew on outdoor steps

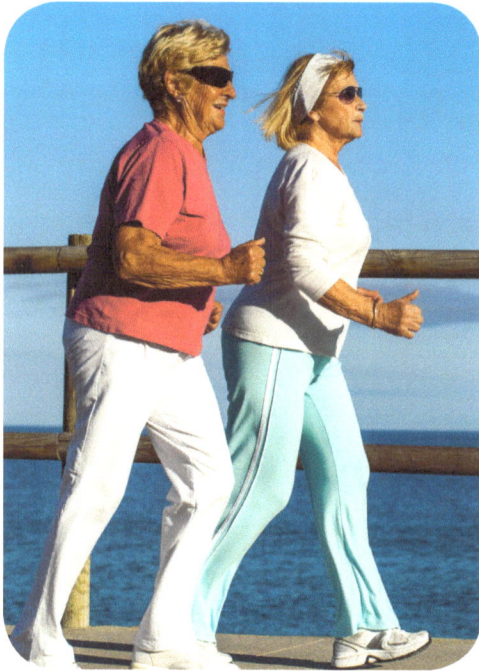

# EXERCISE

When you get home, keep up the exercise program you learned in the hospital. Walking is an important part of your exercise program. It helps to prevent blood clots from forming. A good rule of thumb is to walk every hour. You will regain your strength and endurance as you begin to do your normal daily routine.

# INCISION CARE

Look at your incision each day.

Call your doctor if you notice any of these:

- fever over 100° F/37.8° C
- drainage from incision
- redness around incision
- increased swelling around incision
- chest pain
- chest congestion
- problems with breathing
- calf pain or swelling in your legs

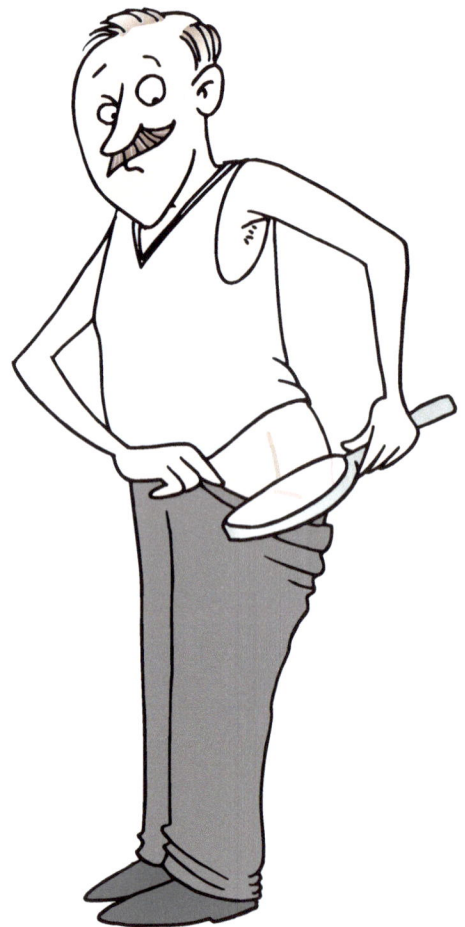

Your staples or stitches will be removed about 10 to 14 days after surgery. Your incision will heal, and the swelling and bruising will get better over the next few weeks.

# SPECIAL EQUIPMENT YOU MAY WANT TO USE AT HOME:

☐ Elastic shoelaces

☐ Back pack, fanny pack, walker basket

☐ Extra cushions, pillows

☐ Walker

☐ Crutches

☐ Cane

☐ Sock donner

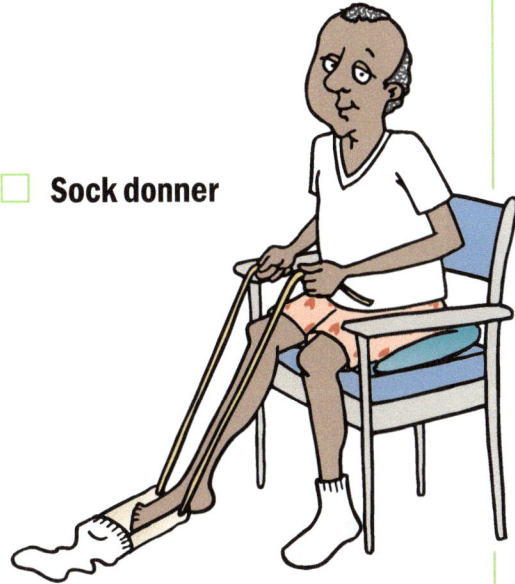

☐ Dressing stick

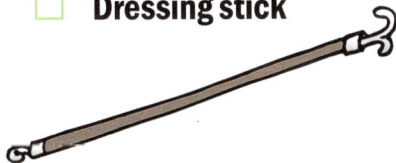

☐ Shoe horn

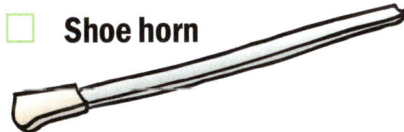

☐ Raised toilet seat

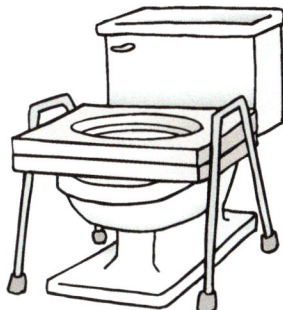

☐ Long-handled sponge

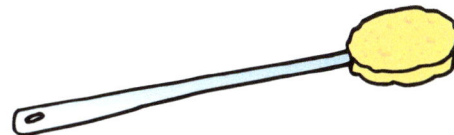

☐ Grabber

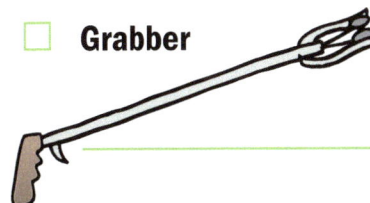

# LIVING WITH YOUR NEW HIP

- **Call your doctor right away**, if you have a fever over 100°F/37.8°C.

- Don't be shy—ask for help when you need it. Your goal is to be able to do things for yourself, but right now you need to take care of your new hip until it fully heals. Do not risk hurting yourself by trying to do too much, too soon.

- Keep your checkup appointment with your doctor. It is important to monitor the healing and function of your new hip.

- To your body, your new hip is a large, foreign substance. Germs from other infections can move to the new hip and cause infection. Call your family doctor at once if you have any signs of infection (urinary tract infection, abscessed teeth, etc.). Early treatment with antibiotics may be needed.

- Tell your dentist and your family doctor BEFORE having your teeth worked on or having any procedure (such as cardiac cath, bladder exam, etc.) or surgery. Antibiotics may be needed before the procedure to prevent infection.

- Your new hip may set off metal detectors, such as those found in airports and some buildings. Your doctor can give you an ID card to carry in your wallet.

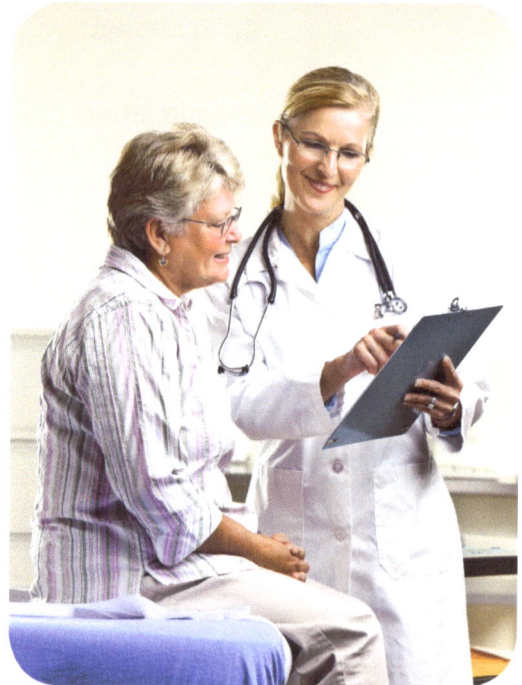

# Your new hip

replacement socket

plastic lining

ball replacement

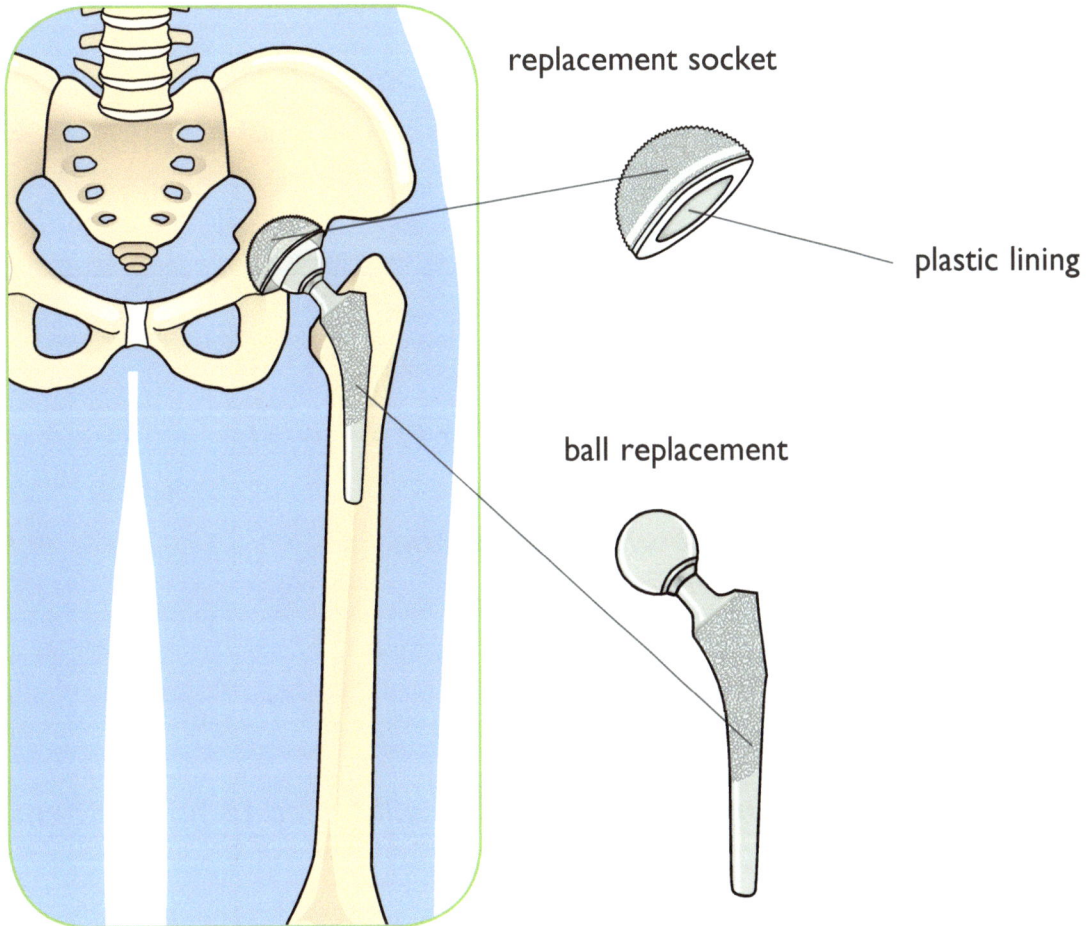

This book is only to help you
learn, and should not be used
to replace any of your doctor's
advice or treatment.

Published and distributed by:
Pritchett & Hull Associates, Inc.

Printed in the U.S.A.

# Points to discuss with your doctor

Take time now while your thoughts are fresh to write down any questions you wish to ask your doctor. Here are a few to help you get started.

*What do you recommend I do to avoid constipation?*

*What type of anesthesia is available?*

*What do you recommend?*

*Should I take my daily medicines on the day of surgery?*

*How long will my family wait while I am in the operating and recovery rooms?*

*How will I get pain relief after surgery?*

*Will I have hip precautions? If so, how long will I need to follow them?*

*When can I drive?*

*When can I have sex?*

*Do I need to take any precautions when having sex?*

*Is there any medical equipment that I should order before surgery?*

www.ingramcontent.com/pod-product-compliance
Lightning Source LLC
Chambersburg PA
CBHW060855270326
41934CB00002B/155